Southeast Indiana Agritourism Guide

Farms, Farmers Markets and Garden Centers

Indiana Consumer Agricultural Guide
Book 1

Paul R. Wonning

Southeast Indiana Agritourism Guide
Published By Paul R. Wonning
Copyright 2017 by Paul R. Wonning
Print Edition

mossyfeetbooks@gmail.com

If you would like email notification of when new Mossy Feet books become available email the author for inclusion in the subscription list.

Mossy Feet Books
www.mossyfeetbooks.com

Indiana Places

http://indianaplaces.blogspot.com/

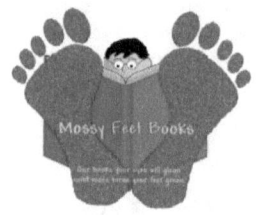

Description

Find the best Farm fresh produce, meats, eggs and plants using the Southeast Indiana Agritourism Guide as your source manual. The guide lists farmers markets, garden centers, nurseries and farms where consumers may purchase local agricultural products.

Table of Contents

Southeast Indiana Agritourism Guide
Paul R. Wonning

History of the Marketplace

Egyptian Market Place

The marketplace dates back to ancient times with the first evidence of markets found in the culture of ancient Egypt. Each Egyptian city and town had a marketplace where people could buy and sell goods. Common agricultural products for sale included barley, emmer wheat, fruit, vegetables, cattle, goats, ducks, geese and flax for making linen. Crafts people sold pottery, sandals, jewelry, furniture and other things they made. Since they did not have money, they used the barter system to purchase goods. The standard measure of weight in Egypt was the deben, which is about three ounces. In each market there was a balancing scale. If you wanted to purchase something, you had to bring something you wanted to trade. When you picked out what you wanted, the merchant placed it on the scale and added metal debens to it until it balanced. You would then place your trade item on the scale and added debens until it balanced. If the two were equal, you traded. If not, you made adjustments to the amount of goods to be bartered until they did and you could complete the sale.

Greek Markets

A large open area occupied the central area of most Greek cities. This area, called the agora, provided a location for merchants to set up their stalls. Greeks of all classes visited this market to purchase silks, spices, fresh fruit, vegetables, fish, meat, linen, ivory and other goods with origins across the Mediterranean Sea region.

Roman Markets

The Romans duplicated the Greek fashion of locating a marketplace near the center of the city. Called a forum, merchants in the marketplace sold a variety of goods that included prepared foods like bread, hot sausages, pastries, and chickpeas. Like the Greek agora, traders also sold silks, spices, fresh fruit, vegetables, fish, meat, linen, ivory and other goods with origins across the Mediterranean Sea region. Signs placed at busy places within the market, like an amphitheater, provided a place for merchants to advertise their wares and locations within the forum. A large city, like Rome, also had bathhouses, circuses, amphitheatres, theatres and other entertainment. The marketplace was generally paved and people entered through large gates. Also in larger cities a separate market, the *macellum*, provided luxury goods and top quality foods for rich residents of a city. Some vendors would visit wealthy people in their homes. In general, though, the forum's visitors included both men and women and citizens from across the economic strata.

Medieval Marketplace

During Medieval times marketplaces generally were located near castles, manors and monasteries. The monarch awarded a charter for these markets, designating a day of the week they could operate. Once a market received a charter, nearby markets could not open on the same day. Weekly or biweekly markets generally offered fresh produce, meat and other necessities. Vendors selling other goods usually crowded around in alleys and side streets. Large cities might have a market operating every day. In addition to merchandise, musicians, jugglers and other entertainers usually frequented the market, performing for tips. Communities along the sea had beach markets where fishermen sold fresh caught fish.

Colonial Farmer's Markets

Massachusetts Royal Governor John Winthrop ordered the opening of the first farmers market in colonial America. This was an open air market and would remain so until 1662. In that year the market constructed a wooden building to shelter the merchants and customers.

Great Country Store

The General Court of Connecticut decreed that the town of Hartford should establish a public market in 1643. Called the Great Country Store, the market took place on every Wednesday the site of the Old State House, on the southeast corner of Meeting House Yard. Vendors sold all manner of merchandise at the market from fresh produce to cattle to any type of merchandise.

Pennsylvania

Philadelphia opened a public market in 1693. This market opened twice a week on High Street, which was renamed Market Street. Forty miles to the north, the village of Easton in Pennsylvania opened a public market in 1752. Billed as "America's Longest Continuous Running Open-Air Market," this market has remained open since its inception. It was one of three places in the new United States where the Declaration of Independence was first read publicly. The market is right on the banks of the Delaware River, centered between New York City, Philadelphia, and Trenton, New Jersey. Still running after all these years, it is one of the five oldest continuously running farmers markets in the world. For more information, contact:

Easton Farmers' Market

Saturdays: 9am – 1pm

Historic Centre Square, Downtown Easton

https://eastonfarmersmarket.com/

Markets Importance

The farmer's market provided a valuable place for urban dwellers to purchase their foods and served as the primary source for farm products. The farmers sold a variety of foodstuffs. Fresh vegetables were limited to whatever was in season, however the vegetables that stored well like including corn meal, onions, potatoes, apples, sauerkraut, pickles and dried fruit were available year round.

Decline of the Farmer's Markets

Over time, the cities grew in size, pushing the farmers that grew the food away from the city center. The farmers began shipping their food over longer distances. When the railways emerged in the 1850's as a major transportation medium, remote markets not available before opened to farmers. During the early part of the Twentieth Century the first supermarkets emerged. As supermarkets and a mass food distribution system evolved, interest in farmer's markets declined and many markets disappeared.

Reemergence

A resurgence of interest in locally produced food beginning in the 1970's created a gradual increase in markets across the United States. By the 1990's the numbers of farmers markets began a strong increase in numbers and by 2006 almost three million Americans purchased products at a local farmer's market. Today the number of farmers markets has increased and many smaller cities and towns have established markets in their town squares where local farmers, artisans and other crafts people can sell their goods and produce.

Clark County

Davis Nursery & Country Market

Established in 1985 near Indiana State Road 62 in New Washington, Indiana with two greenhouses, the Davis family's greenhouse operation grew to include five greenhouses in 1990. That year a tornado leveled the operation. After the total loss of the greenhouses and stock, the family built four gutter-connected greenhouses on a property they owned across the road, Davis Implement Incorporated. The new company, Davis Nursery, sold plants wholesale to Field's Produce in Madison and later to several greenhouse operations across the river in Louisville, Kentucky. The company also sold plants to a growing stream of retail customers at its facility in New Washington, allowing it to grow to sixteen greenhouses.

Davis Nursery & Country Market

Two of Davis' main customers, Fields Produce in Madison and Ed's Fruit Market in Jeffersonville Indiana, decided to close in 2003 and 2004 respectively, and the Davis family decided to buy both businesses. They established the Davis Nursery & Country Market in 2004. Currently the company operates a twenty greenhouse growing facility at their New Washington location as a growing facility and sells plants, nursery stock and fresh produce at its retail locations in Jeffersonville and Madison. The company purchases fresh produce from local growers as well as other sources to have fresh, quality produce available at its stores year round. The company provides products for Boar's Head Premium Deli Meats & Cheeses delis and stocks European Import Specialty Food and Stonewall Kitchen products in their stores.

Places customers can find Davis Nursery and Country Market

Davis Nursery & Country Market

1708 E 10th St

Jeffersonville, Indiana 47130

Davis Nursery & Country Market

812-284-3283

202 Clifty Dr

Madison, Indiana 47250

812-273-1288

Davis Nursery & Country Market - Home

www.davisnurserycountrymarket.com/

HB Farms and Greenhouses

Established in 2000, this family owned farm produced vegetables for sale at local farmer's markets and a fall offering of pumpkins, gourds and mums. They grew the mums in the ground and dug them just prior to sale, which they displayed on a local highway visible to travelers on their way to a local attraction. They sold 2500 mums and their crop of pumpkins grown on three acres. The second year HB Farms expanded the production to 12,500 mums, mostly grown in pots, and ten acres of pumpkins. The potted mums enabled them to develop a wholesale market. The business continued to grow and today HB Farms produces over 70,000 mums, including over 100 varieties and a full palette of colors. The selection includes 8" pots, 11" hanging baskets, and 12" Patio Pots. In addition to mums,

HB Farms grows Montauk Daisies, ornamental kale, ornamental cabbage and hardy asters.

Spring Offerings

HB Farms specialized in petunias and perennial flowers. They offer over eighty different kinds of perennial flowers and an extensive line of petunias grown in hanging baskets and patio pots.

Robert J. Wimsatt

HB Farms and Greenhouses

8400 Scottsville Rd.

Borden, IN 47106

Phone: 502-296-9493

contact@hbfarmsgreenhouses.com

http://www.hbfarmsgreenhouses.com

Huber Orchard and Winery

German immigrant Simon Huber founded Huber Orchard and Winery in 1843. From his native Baden-Baden, Germany, Simon learned the winemaking craft and brought his knowledge with him to his 80 acre farm. He made his first wines from strawberries. The farm prospered and grew through seven generation and has grown to over 600 acres. The Huber Orchard and Winery is the largest winemaking operation in Indiana. The eighteen varieties of grapes produce over 400,000 pounds of grapes on average per year. The farm produces more than wine. The product mix includes fruits and vegetables. The Huber's Starlight Distillery on the farm produces different kinds of brandies. Tours are available for those wishing to learn more.

For more information, contact:

Huber Orchard and Winery

19816 Huber Rd

Borden, IN 47106

812-923-9463

http://www.huberwinery.com

Jeffersonville Farmers Market

This seasonal open air Farmer's Market is located at the corner of Market and Mulberry Streets at the Big Four Bridge in downtown Jeffersonville, Indiana.

The winter market is in the gym of the First Presbyterian Church at the corner of Walnut and Chestnut Streets in Jeffersonville, Indiana.

Dates

Saturdays, 9am - noon

Tuesdays, 3 - 6pm

May - October

Saturdays, 9:30am - noon

November - May

Jeffersonville, Indiana 47130.

812-283-0301

http://farmersmarketonline.com/fm/JeffersonvilleFarmers Market.html

https://www.facebook.com/Clark-County-Farmers-Market-at-Jeffersonville-350542722688/

Joe Huber's Family Farm and Restaurant

Inspired by a bumper crop of green beans, Joseph H. Huber Jr. advertised the crop as a "pick your own," proposition to customers in the local newspaper in 1967. When townspeople began flocking to the farm to pick the beans, Huber and his family were surprised to discover that these urbanites thought picking their own vegetables was a fun way to spend an afternoon. The vision of Joe Huber's Family Farm and Restaurant sprang into being.

Joe Huber (March 21, 1955 - July 27, 2015)

The son of Joseph H. Huber Jr. and Bonnie Kruer Huber, Joe was native to Starlight, Indiana. Huber grew up on the family farm and attended Flaget High School, graduating in 1973. He attended Purdue University, graduating with a agricultural economics degree in 1977. He married Kathryn M. "Kathy" Kirchgessner in 1974, with whom he would have three children. Kathryn passed away in 2008.

The Beginning

Joe and Bonnie purchased the 200 acre farm after his father passed away. His father, Joseph H. Huber Sr. had initially purchased the farm in 1926. They housed many of the farm workers on the farm with Mary providing home cooked meals for them. Mary had dressed the chickens, and the children milked cows. Joseph Sr. passed away in 1967, after which Joseph and Bonnie purchased the farm. The produce, livestock and other products from the farm provided food for the eleven children and produced the income needed to raise the growing family.

Joe Huber's Family Farm and Restaurant

Shortly after the experiment with the excess green beans, the family transformed their garage into a farm market. Shortly after this they built the Farm Market. They opened the restaurant in 1983, using Mary's family and farm worker tested recipes as the foundation of the fare served in the restaurant. Consisting of chicken and dumplings, fried chicken, mashed potatoes and gravy, a variety of fresh vegetables from the garden, homemade rolls, fresh fruit pies, the menu proved a hit.

Huber's Orchard, Winery, and Vineyards

The tradition continues, with the restaurant serving the same types of food cooked by Mary for the children and the "pick your own" fruits and vegetables providing food and entertainment for their customers.

Joe Huber's Family Farm and Restaurant

2421 Engle Road

Starlight, Indiana 47106

(812) 923-5255

http://www.joehubers.com

McCoy's Nursery

Established in 1969, McCoy's Nursery is a garden center, greenhouse, nursery and landscape company located near Charlestown, Indiana. The garden center offers an extensive line of annuals, biennials, perennials, veggies and herbs, and nursery stock. Landscape services include both residential and commercial landscape design and installation.

McCoy's Nursery

8911 Highway 62

Charlestown, IN 47111-8407

http://www.mccoysnursery.com

(812) 256-4769

Old Thyme Log House Garden

Founded in 1997 near Otisco, Indiana the Old Thyme Loghouse Garden grows vegetable, annual flowers, herb and perennial flower transplants.

Old Thyme Loghouse Garden

8207 Old State Road 3

Otisco, IN 47163-9456Map

(812) 256-7971

http://www.oldthymeloghousegarden.com

Walnut Ridge Nursery & Garden Center

History

Walnut Hill was first established as J Julius' Sons in 1913, after William M. Julius purchased a nine acre property on Hamburg Pike. The business included several greenhouses, a potting shed, a boiler and a house. A tunnel connected the house and the greenhouse operation. The next year the operation produced cut flowers and bedding plants. The family opened J Julius' Sons Florist in downtown Jeffersonville, Indiana that same year, 1914. William's younger brother Louis managed the florist business while William M and another brother, Edmund, operated the greenhouse. They continued to sell bedding plants from the Hamburg Pike location for the next several years. A fire at the Indiana State Prison in Jefferson in 1918 caused state officials to close it and build a new facility at Pendleton, Indiana. When the prison closed, the Julius family purchased the greenhouse in 1921 and moved it to their Hamburg Pike property. In 1929 the family purchased another greenhouse operation in Clarksville, adding its two greenhouses to its operation. The 1937 Ohio River Flood covered the florist shop in Jeffersonville with flood waters and threatened to flood the Hamburg Pike operation. In 1952 the family split the florist business from the greenhouse business. The greenhouse business became Walnut Ridge Greenhouses while the florist remained J Julius' Sons Florist. Walnut Ridge Greenhouses began selling wholesale in 1953 and opened Walnut Ridge Garden Center in the fall of the same year. Growth continued in 1960 with the opening of a second garden center in New Albany. During this era the operation expanded its offerings to include trees, shrubs and Christmas decor. From 1963 until 1968 the company operated two temporary greenhouses to sell plants in satellite operations. The company added landscape design to its services in 1964. By 1984 the company had two garden centers, a thriving landscape design service and two acres under glass that produced several million plants annually. Walnut Ridge Pool and Patio split off the business in 1990 and Walnut Ridge Greenhouses established Ridge Wholesale Nursery to sell trees and shrubs to garden centers in the surrounding areas.

Today Walnut Ridge Nursery and Garden Center offers many more products in addition to landscaping, plants and garden supplies. These include:

Apparel & Accessories

Dishware and Home Accessories

Outdoor Decor

Lawn Care

Gardening Supplies

Plants & Flowers

Annuals

Grasses

Groundcovers

Perennials

Plants & Flowers Miscellaneous

Pre-potted Containers & Urns

Trees, Shrubs & Roses

Weeks Roses

Tropical Houseplants

Seasonal Plants

Vines & Climbers

Home & Garden Supplies

Gifts

Seasonal Items

Walnut Ridge Nursery & Garden Center

2108 Hamburg Pike

Jeffersonville, IN 47130 US

https://walnutridge.com

Clark-Floyd Counties Convention-Tourism

315 Southern Indiana Avenue

Jeffersonville IN 47130

http://gosoin.com

812-282-6654

tourism@GoSoIN.com

Dearborn County

Abundant Green Pastures Farm

Since 2006 Abundant Green Pastures Farm has provided healthy, tasty grass fed beef and pork for consumers that enjoy healthy, flavorful meat.

Healthy Grass Fed Beef

Most beef on the market today is from grain fed Black Angus cattle, produced on large feed lots. Abundant Green Pastures Farm has taken a different tack, using a breed of cattle called Red Devon because of the quality of their meat and their ability to adapt to changing weather conditions in open pasture. Using a type of breeding called closed herd, the farm has built a herd of healthy cattle in which they control the genetics because they do not introduce cattle from outside the farm to breed. The breed has been in America since early colonial times, first introduced by the Pilgrims sometime after 1620. Using pasture land that has a rich blend of grasses and legumes, the farm produces a tasty, high quality, healthy meat. The farm utilized a system of ponds and a fifteen acre lake to irrigate the pasture, when necessary, to keep it healthy and growing.

Healthy Pastured Pork

Using the same closed herd type of breeding, Abundant Green Pastures Farm produced pasture fed pigs that receive 80% of their calories from pasture and tree nuts and 20% from non-GMO grain. Farrowing (pregnant) sows have their own pasture, farrowing hut and water supply to protect the health of the piglets. The producers use no antibiotics in the production of any of their animals.

Abundant Green Pastures Farm

1165 Chapelow Ridge Road

West Harrison, Indiana 47060

812-637-3039

www.abundantgreenpastures.com

Beiersdorfer Orchard

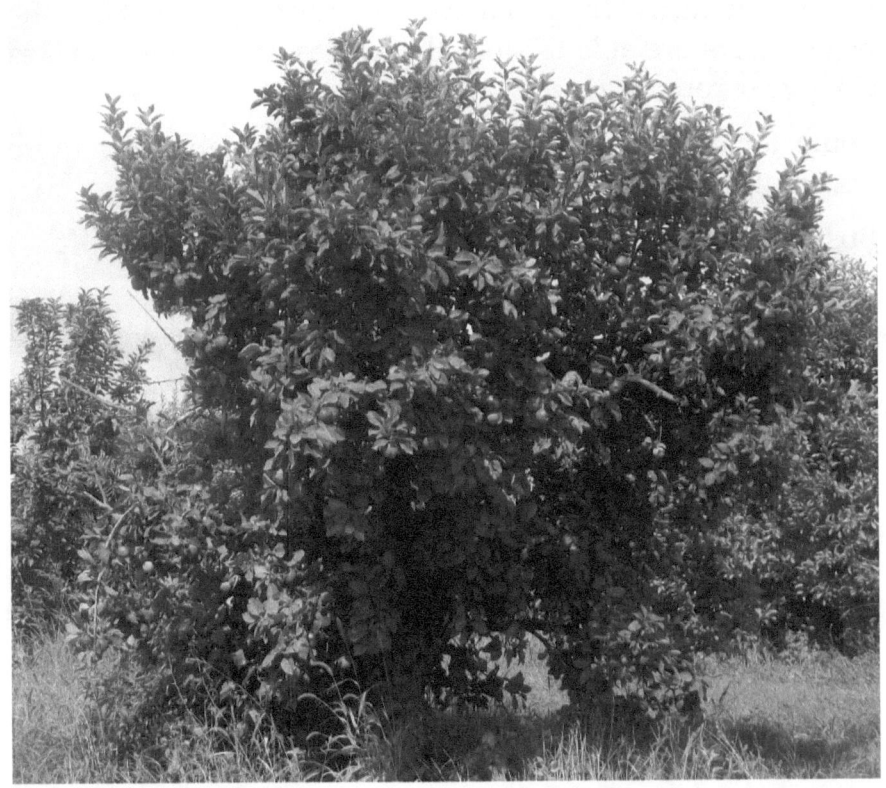

Beiersdorfer Orchard is a family owned business operating in Southeastern Indiana.

While specializing in apples and apple cider, we have wide selection of mouth-watering fruits such as peaches, pears, plums, etc. to fill your needs.

We cater to everyone, from the casual individual shopper to commercial customers.

Guilford

Located on 75 acres in Guilford, Beiersdorfer Orchard is owned and operated by Hilda Beiersdorfer and family. Here you will find rows and rows of fruit trees where the apples are picked and washed before selling. Some are processed into cider and apple butter. The farm market has a variety of items for sale, including homegrown apples, peaches and plums, along with products for canning. Because the Beierdorfers are able to store the apples, the orchard makes cider year-round.

Tours for children and adults are also available. For more information call 812-487-2695.

Business Hours at Beiersdorfer Orchard:

Monday - Saturday, 9 am - 6 pm

Sunday, 1 pm - 6 pm

Beiersdorfer Orchard

21874 Kuebel Road

Guilford, IN 47022

Phone: 812-487-2695

http://www.beiersdorferorchard.com/

https://www.facebook.com/pages/Beiersdorfer-Orchard/179950802084149

Bright Farmers Market

Meet your farming and crafting neighbors on State Line Road, in Bright every Friday, 3 - 6:30

May thru mid - October

812-623-8184

https://www.facebook.com/farmersmarketbright/

Busse Fruit and Vegetable Farm

Busse's Farm offers a wide variety of bedding plants for purchase, including 19 different varieties of tomatoes, peppers, zucchini, eggplant and herbs. In the fall, choose from approximately 2,500 pumpkins and 500 gourds, or pick from the farm's vast selection of mums.

Busse Fruit and Vegetable Farm also offers a wide variety of fresh, locally grown fruits and vegetables grown on their farm above Aurora.

Busse's Farm usually recommends that you call before coming to ensure they are open.

Busse Farm

7096 State Route 48

Aurora, IN 47001

812-926-1807

https://www.facebook.com/Busses-Fruit-and-Vegetable-Farm-255222574495199/

Dillsboro Farmers Market

Heritage Pointe at North & Bank Streets

Dillsboro, Indiana 47018

(812) 432-3243

https://www.facebook.com/Dillsboro-Farmers-Market-1682514815354955/

Greystone Family Farm

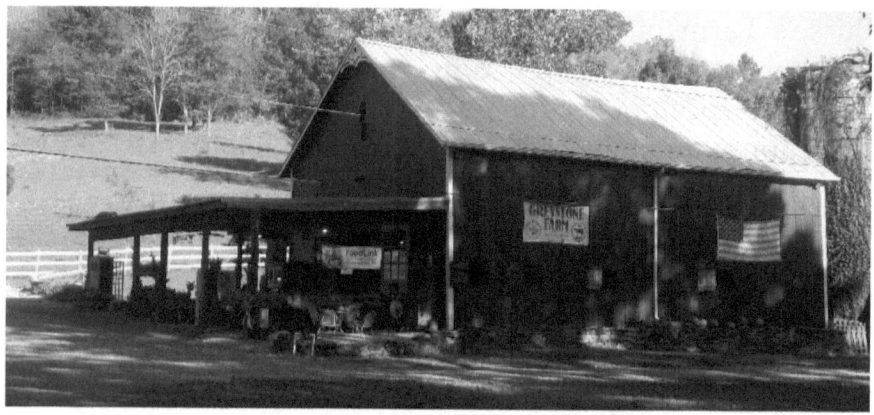

Greystone Farm supplies a variety of high quality and locally grown produce. This is a family farm, owned and operated by Kelly and Adam Young.

Fall farm items for sale are corn stalks, straw, gourds, carving pumpkins, pie pumpkins, mini pumpkins, Indian corn and more. Other items that come from a few local farms include Beiersdorfer's apple cider, apple and pumpkin butter and apples from Crosby Orchard.

Springtime selections include buckwheat and alfalfa/clover honey, green onions, herb plants, free-range chickens and Tennessee tomatoes.

The farm also produces beef, pork, chickens, rabbits, brown eggs and local honey. Seasonal produce includes a variety of peppers (hot and sweet), eggplant, potatoes, yams, beets, turnips, cabbage, candy onions, acorn squash, pears and string beans.

Business hours:

Open Daily from May 1 through October 31

By Appointment during the off season

Greystone Farm

15412 Wilson Creek Road

Lawrenceburg, IN 47025

812-926-2132

greystonefamilyfarm@gmail.com

https://www.greystonefamilyfarm.com/

http://www.facebook.com/greystonefamilyfarm

Lawrenceburg Farmers Market

The Lawrenceburg Farmers Market is a seasonal open air market with vendors that offer fresh produce, jams, jellies, plants, flowers, eggs, honey, baked good, soaps, lotions and more. It is located in Newtown Park along US route 50 between Main and Park Street in Lawrenceburg, Indiana.

Dates

Saturdays, 9am - 1pm

June - mid-October

Lawrenceburg Farmers Market

(812) 537-4507

https://www.facebook.com/events/downtown-lawrenceburg-farmers-market-kick-off/1664241777219089/

Lobenstein's Farm

Located in the northern part of Dearborn County, Lobenstein's Farm is home to one of Southeastern Indiana's largest pumpkin festivals. The annual festival is held the first three weekends in October and draws about 30,000 people annually. Visitors are able to pick their own pumpkins from the field, enjoy hayrides, craft booths and a petting zoo. Lobenstein's Farm is located in St. Leon approximately 30 miles from Cincinnati and three miles from I-74. For more information and directions to Lobenstein's Farm, call 812-576-3177.

Lobenstein's Farm

29703 Post Road

St. Leon, IN 47032

812-576-3177

https://www.facebook.com/Lobenstein-Farm-115504615177718/

McCabe's Greenhouse & Floral

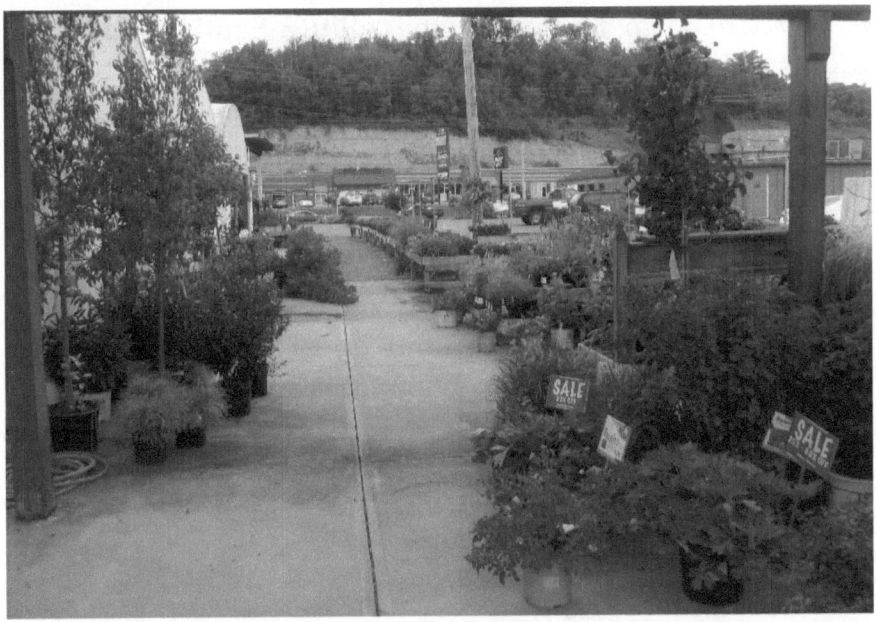

McCabe's Greenhouse & Floral offers customers a full garden center stocked with plants, many of which they produce in their extensive range of greenhouses, and gardening supplies that can fill your every gardening need. The floral shop provides arrangements for weddings, funerals and other events. The gift shop stocks home decor, garden gifts and specialized gifts that can serve your personal needs. McCabes' also has a full line of homemade fudge available in a host of flavors.

McCabe's Greenhouse & Floral

1066 W Eads Pkwy

Lawrenceburg, IN 47025

(812) 537-4525

https://mccabesgreenhouseandfloral.com/

Mt. Tabor Alpaca Farm

An 89-acre farm located in the rolling Southeast Indiana countryside, Mt. Tabor Alpaca Farm is a great destination for groups of all ages! This popular agri-tourism spot is home to a large herd of alpacas, the gentle animals prized for the super-soft fiber. Somewhat similar to llama in appearance, domesticated alpacas are originally from South America and live in herds. Enjoy a special behind-the-scenes tour of this scenic farm, where you will learn more about these magnificent animals and meet the farm's other inhabitants, including goats, honeybees and horses.

Tour - $5 adults, $2 children

Advance reservations required

812-926-3732.

Mt. Tabor Alpaca Farm

9267 Mt. Tabor Road

Aurora, IN 47001

Phone: 812-926-3732

1-513-200-4166 - Toll Free

http://www.mttaboralpacas.com

https://www.facebook.com/mttaboralpacas

Phillips Berry Patch

The Very Berry Patch can be found at 9429 York Ridge Road in New Alsace. Owners James and Darlene Phillips have a variety of items depending on season, including berries, pumpkins, gourds and mums. Business hours at The Very Berry Patch vary according to season, so you may wish to call before visiting. For further information or directions, call 812-623-1433.

Phillips Berry Patch

9429 York Ridge Road

New Alsace, IN

Phone: 812-623-1433

https://www.facebook.com/phillipsberrypatch

Randolph's Family Farm

Randolph's Family Farm is a 55 acre farm located in Southeast Indiana near Dillsboro. The Randolph's raise and grow their own food and pasture their animals as natural as possible and without any antibiotics, hormones or chemicals. The family bought the farm in 2016 and considers it the best thing they ever did with raising our two girls. They also have a family milk cow named Ginger that gives them fresh A2/A2 Jersey Milk & Cream. With that they also make our own ice cream and butter. The family has chickens and ducks for eggs and they believe that there is nothing like a farm fresh egg. We also like to provide for others. The owner says that she won't eat it or drink it she doesn't expect others to. The family has added honeybees to their farm. The owner loves working with my bees and loves the honey they produce. They don't use any chemicals on our farm and never will. They have two ponds that the girls love to fish in and they have some pretty bass and bluegills. They also raise our own hay for our farm animals. So this farm is not just a hobby farm but its becoming a nice big working farm. They sell to the public items that they raise and produce on our farm. You can never eat as good as you can when it comes fresh from the farm, especially when it's natural and raised properly. Please find and like their page on FB. They are always adding new stuff to the farm.

513-520-4634

randolphsfarm@yahoo.com

https://www.facebook.com/randolphsfarm

Riehle's Select Gourmet Popcorn

Riehle's Select Gourmet Popcorn is a family owned and operated farm that produces top quality gourmet popcorn. They offer thirteen specialty varieties of mouthwatering, whole grain, gourmet popcorn including our virtually hull-free popcorn, ladyfinger hulless microwave popcorn and organic popcorn. Order their products on on their website.

Riehle's Select Popcorn

Riehle Enterprise, LLC

9632 N. County Rd. 800 East

Sunman, IN 47041

812-623-8172

Gourmet popcorn

https://www.selectpopcorn.com

https://www.facebook.com/riehles.select.gourmet.popping
.corn/?ref=br_rs

Salatin's Orchard

Donna and Richard Salatin started their orchard in 1984 as a hobby. It has since grown into a full-time business. Located on Chesterville Road in Moores Hill, Salatin's Orchard grows and sells twenty-four varieties of apples. The Salatins also make their own cider. Apples that have fallen on the ground, however, are never used for cider or sold. Instead, the fallen apples are donated to the Red Wolf Sanctuary in Dillsboro to feed the bears that live there.

Business hours at Salatin's Orchard:

Monday-Sunday, 10 AM - 7 PM.

Berries, pears, winter squash, honey and apple butter also are grown or produced and sold at Salatin's, depending on season. To learn more, or to find out about taking a tour, call Donna or Richard at 812-744-3481.

Salatin's Orchard

10514 Chesterville Road

Moores Hill, IN 47032-9255

812-744-3481

https://www.facebook.com/Salatins-Orchard-111522905561999/

Small Acres Farm

Small Acres Farm sells top quality vegetables at local farmer's markets and at their farm. See the hours posted on their website.

23006 Kammeyer Rd.

Sunman, IN 47041

https://www.facebook.com/smallacresfamilyfarm/

W.J. Strassell & Sons

Strassell Greenhouses offer a complete line of bedding plants, hanging baskets and fall mums. Friendly, Clean, and Affordable plants

W.J. Strassell & Sons

7748 E County Road 50 N

Moores Hill, Indiana 47032

(812) 744-5115

Open · Closes 7PM

https://www.facebook.com/WJ-Strassell-and-Sons-Inc-1483355598549022/

Dearborn County Visitor Center

320 Walnut Street

Lawrenceburg, IN 47025

http://www.visitsoutheastindiana.com

812-537-0814

Decatur County

Gauck's Meats

Pork Products

Grass Fed Beef

Pasture Raised Chickens

Gauck's Meats uses no artificial growth hormones or antibiotics on their livestock. They also offer farm fresh eggs.

Gaucks Meats

6472 E County Road 300 N

Greensburg, IN 47240

812-614-1223

https://www.facebook.com/pages/category/Local-Business/Gauck-Family-Livestock-156634704385463/

kimmiegauck@hotmail.com

Harper Valley Farms

Established in 1941, Harper Valley Farms offers fresh farm grown beef, pork and eggs. The farm also grows a wide variety of vegetables for sale at local farmer's markets or directly from the farm. Vegetables include tomatoes, sweet corn, cabbage, peppers, broccoli, melons, strawberries, cauliflower, pumpkins, squash and gourds. Customers may also rent Grandma Pearcy's Hilltop Rental Home as a weekend getaway. In the fall the farm operates a pumpkin patch where customers may pick their own pumpkins. Customers may also buy ready picked pumpkins, get lost in a sunflower maze or purchase a beautiful fall mum.

For more information, contact:

Harper Valley Farms

13094 South County Road 600 West

Westport, Indiana 47283

812 591 3416

www.harpervalleyfarms.com

https://www.facebook.com/indianapumpkinpatch/

Pumpkin Patch Harper Valley

www.indianapumpkinpatch.com

Highpoint Orchard and Farm Market

The Highpoint Orchard and Farm Market features a unique farm market featuring fresh-baked goods, produce, antiques, gifts, apples and other fruits and vegetables when in season. A peaceful, relaxing country setting on one of the highest geographic points in Decatur, so you have a good veiw of the surrounding countryside as you shop the 25 varieties of apples, fresh local produce and the gift shop.

Highpoint Orchard and Farm Market

3321 N Old Hwy. 421

Greensburg, IN 47240

812.663.9534

http://www.highpointorchard.com

Vanderburs Greenhouse

Becky (Beesley) and David Vanderbur established Vanderburs Greenhouse in 1998. The company offers a large selection of potted plants, perennials, hanging baskets, annuals, and garden plants and seeds.

Vanderburs Greenhouse

5325 W County Road 800 S

Greensburg, Indiana 47240

(812) 591-2557

https://www.facebook.com/Vanderburs-Greenhouse-287894868030/

Vohland Nursery

Established in 1930, Vohland Nursery provides it customers with a wide variety of plants and services. These include:

Annuals

Perennials

Shrubs

Trees

Water Feature Design and Equipment

Stonework

Landscape Design

Vohland Nursery

2085 Moscow Rd

Greensburg, Indiana 47240

(812) 663-7773

http://www.vohlandnursery.com

https://www.facebook.com/vohlandnursery/

Visit Decatur County, Inc.

211 N Broadway St

Greensburg, IN 47240

http://www.visitgreensburg.com/

Franklin County

Brookville Farmers' Market

The Brookville Farmer's Market generally opens the third week of May on Main Street (US 52) on the south side of town in a grassy area on the west side of the highway just north of Pearl Street. Market hours are from 3:30 until about 7:00 PM. Expect to find handmade crafts, produce, baked goods and plants for sale.

Brookville Farmers' Market

110 Main Street

Brookville, IN 47012

765-265-6115

http://www.localharvest.org/brookville-farmers-market-M21857

https://www.facebook.com/groups/63096253830/about/

Colorworks Greenhouse

Colorworks Greenhouse offers annuals, perennials, hanging baskets, potted plants and ornamentals at their greenhouse on Holland Road. Fall offerings include mums, ornamental cabbage and pansies. The company also sells wholesale quantities to nurseries and garden centers.

Colorworks Greenhouse

8080 Holland Rd.

Brookville, Indiana 47012

https://www.facebook.com/colrwrks/

Doll's Orchards, LLC

Established by Adam and Anna Weber when they purchased the property on February 28, 1924, the Sisters of St. Francis purchased the property and orchard on September 19, 1930. The Sisters of St. Francis used the apples in the kitchen of the Motherhouse Convent in Oldenburg. The Sisters sold the orchard to the George Doll family, who already owned and operated an orchard nearby, in 1970. Originally the orchard produced only apples; however the Dolls have added thornless blackberries, peaches and many varieties of apples not formerly grown.

Located just off Indiana State Road 229 on Tony Road, about four miles south of Peppertown and just outside of Oldenburg, Dolls Orchard opens in the fall when the apples ripen. Visitors may purchase many varieties of apples, apple cider and other products at the orchard. For more information, contact:

Doll's Orchards

21134 Tony Rd

Batesville, IN 47006

Phone: (812) 934-4563

http://oldenburgapplelady.com

https://www.facebook.com/DollsOrchard/

Michaela Farm

Sister Michaela Lindemann, one of the first sisters to join the Sisters of St. Francis in 1851, is the namesake of Michaela Farm. Sister Micheala took charge of the newly acquired 40 acres of land in Franklin County in 1854. In the beginning the farm produced food for local orphans whose parents had died during a cholera epidemic that the Sisters at the convent had agreed to take care of. The farm produced food for the Academy of the Immaculate Conception in Oldenburg. Products included cattle, hogs and chickens as well as butter, egg and cream. The orchards produced fruit, jams and jellies. In 2004 the Sisters established Michaela Farm and completed some extensive renovation projects. Still owned by the Oldenburg Sisters of St. Francis, the farm no longer has cattle on the farm, however they do maintain their own flock of chickens. The Farm welcomes volunteers to work at various tasks. The store is open from 8:00 a.m. to dusk and is located in the old office. The farm sells honey, eggs, fresh produce (in season), a variety of nuts, dried herbs and Doll's Orchard jelly and applesauce. CSA programs available for customers. The huge barn, known locally as the "Cow Barn," is reportedly the largest barn in Franklin County.

Michaela Farm

3127 IN-229

Batesville, IN 47006

(812) 933-0661

https://oldenburgfranciscans.org/michaela-farm/

https://www.facebook.com/Michaelafarm/

Villa Orchard

This is a family owned orchard just outside Oldenburg, Indiana. The orchard opens in early October selling apples, apple butter and cider. Get there fast, as they tend to sell out early.

The Sister's of St. Francis were the first owners of the farm and built the farm house, called St. Clara Villa, in 1896. They used the home as a summer home for children that attended the Academy of the Immaculate Conception in Oldenburg during the summer months. They established the orchard in 1918. The apples they planted many consider heirloom varieties now. The Sisters sold the orchard portion of the farm to Tony Doll, John Eckstein and George Doll in 1970. The Sisters had grown grain crops and raised cattle on what had originally been a 116 acre farm, as well as apples and other fruit crops. The partnership dissolved in the mid to late 1980's, when the partners divided the farm in half, with one half becoming Dolls Orchard. Dave and Judy Eckstein purchased the farm from their parents, John and Julie Eckstein, in 2017. The orchard produces several varieties of heirloom apples as well as Red and Yellow Delicious. They also grow Honey Crisp and Fuji apples and produce honey from bees kept on the farm. In autumn they sell pumpkins they have grown.

Villa Orchard

3301 IN-229

Batesville, IN 47006

(812) 934-2473

Villa Orchard

https://www.facebook.com/The-Villa-Orchard-1500272676872532/

Wendell Farms

Established in 1973, Wendell Farms' main crops are corn, soybeans and wheat. In addition to this, they produce pumpkins and fall mums. They also maintain a petting farm that includes pigs, calves, sheep, goats, horses, donkeys, llamas, alpacas, chickens, ducks, guineas, peacocks, rabbits, a turkey and a goose. The farm opens to the public in early September and continues its hours until October 31. Visitors can pick their own pumpkin, visit the animals in the petting farm, get lost in a corn or straw maze or enjoy any one of several other fun activities. These include:

Corn Maze

Straw Maze

Petting Farm

Farm Land

Education Center

Vegetable Patch

Corn Box

Trike Track

Corn Hole

Tumbling Tubes

Pedal Carts

Combine

Play Area

Duck Races

The farm is open by appointment only at other times. For their current hours, check the web site or Facebook Page.

Wendel Farms

Philip & Susann Wendel, owners

8134 N. State Line Road

Brookville, IN 47012

Call us at 812-775-9051

http://www.wendelfarms.com

https://www.facebook.com/WendelFarms

White Tail Acres Tree Farm

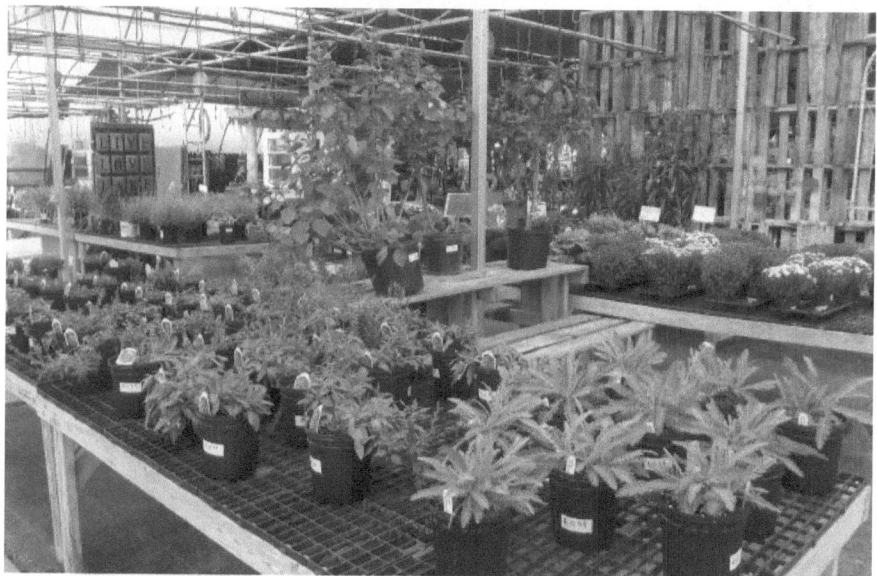

Established in 1984 as a Christmas tree farm, Whitetail Acres has evolved into full service garden center and landscape company. The garden center offers:

Top quality flowers, shrubs & trees

Landscape accessories

Garden art supplies and solutions

Fountains, statuary and pottery

Tropicals and house plants

Lawn care supplies

Home & garden gift shop

Landscaping services include:

Lawn Maintenance

Landscape Maintenance

Seeding & Sod Installation

Paver and wall installation

The tree nursery offers dozens of varieties of hardwood, softwood, fruit and ornamental trees and shrubs.

Christmas Tree Farm

Open from around Thanksgiving until just before Christmas, the Christmas tree farm offers:

Saws for cut-your-own

Tree shaking and baling

Tree drilling

Cozy bonfire

Hayrides through the fields and cut tree pickup

Real Christmas trees!

Free refreshments

Fresh wreaths & roping made daily

Fresh Pre-Cut Beautiful Fraser Firs up to 11-12'

Reindeer Experience And Christmas Tree Farm

9127 Cooley Road

Brookville, IN 47012

White Tail Acres Tree Farm offers wholesale pricing to retailers.

White Tail Acres Tree Farm

8001 Old Blue Creek Rd.

Brookville, IN 47012

765-647-6812

http://www.whitetailacrestreefarm.com

http://www.whitetailacrestreefarm.com/about-us.html

Whites Market Flea Market

Whites Market is both an Indoor and outdoor flea market. Many vendors sell fresh fruit, vegetables and other farm products. If you can think of it, you will find it at White's Flea Market east of Brookville Indiana just off of US 52.

Whites Market Flea Market

3028 Holland Rd

Brookville, IN 47012

(765) 647-3574

https://www.facebook.com/WhitesFarm1922/

http://www.whiteswebsite.com

Franklin County Convention, Recreation and Visitors Commission

P.O. Box 97

Brookville, IN 47012

765-647-6522

http://www.franklincountyin.com/

Jefferson County

Beaver Creek Nursery

Beaver Creek Nursery was founded in 1999. Aside from being the largest retail nursery in Southeastern Indiana, it is also unlike any other nursery you have ever seen. At Beaver Creek Nursery you can not only find almost any plant that is hardy to the area but also relax and enjoy the beautiful serenity of it all. You can take a walk on paths that meander along a creek, through meadows, around a lake, or just stroll around the landscaped gardens.

Beaver Creek Nursery is located at 5530 West County Road 900 South in Madison, Indiana. We are a relaxing 10 minute drive just north of Madison, Indiana or south of Versailles, Indiana just off U.S. 421.

Beaver Creek Nursery

5530 W County Rd 900 S, Madison, IN 47250

(812) 689-5595

https://beavercreeknurseryin.com

https://www.facebook.com/BeaverCreekNursery.Madison.IN/

Davis Nursery & Country Market

See the Clark County Entry

812-284-3283

202 Clifty Dr

Madison, Indiana 47250

812-273-1288

Davis Nursery & Country Market - Home

www.davisnurserycountrymarket.com/

Madison Farmers' Market

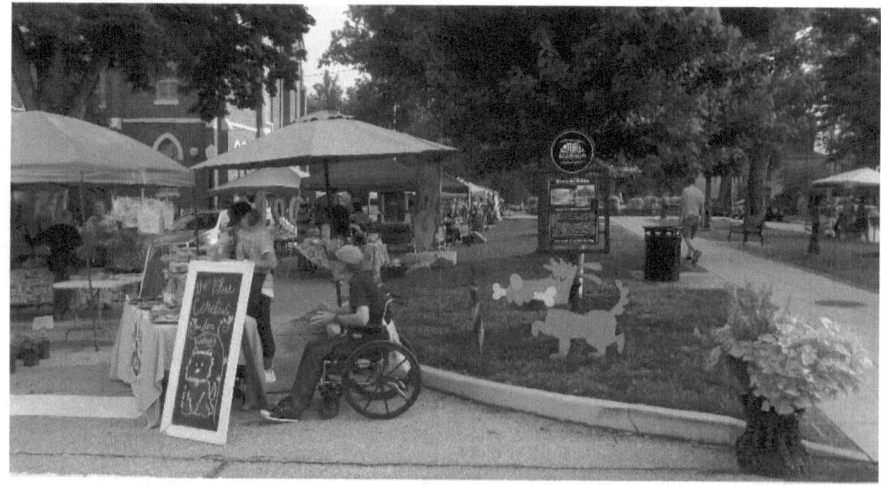

Summer Farmers Market

Broadway Fountain Park

Madison, Indiana 47250

(347) 835-8099

April through October every Saturday from 8 AM to 12 PM at the Broadway Fountain

Winter Market

November through March every Saturday from 9 AM to 12 PM

Trinity United Methodist Church

412 West Main Street,

Madison, IN

Winter Farmers Market

Trinity Church on Broadway Street

412 West Main Street

clerktreasurer@madison-in.gov

(812)265-8313

www.farmersmarketmadison.com

https://www.facebook.com/madison.farmers.market/

River City Nursery

River City Nursery offers large and ornamental trees, shrubs, flowers, hanging baskets and dyed and natural bulk mulch.

Owner: Hannah Ball

3621 Clifty Drive

Madison, Indiana

https://www.facebook.com/rivercitynursery/?__tn__=%2C d%2CP-
R&eid=ARAXy4nD620lMP7k6hdqi9nx0W9BUODKV3Zugu M3ZpNhy2uHpXk9fRuFL4P5IIekl_eNJfGZzfbf--QN

Rykers Ridge Blueberry

We are a small "u-pick" farm who uses all natural processes to grow and harvest over 1000 Blueberry plants during the summer months in Southern Indiana.

Rykers Ridge Blueberry

1492 N Rykers Ridge Rd

Madison, Indiana 47250

(812) 493-5771

https://www.facebook.com/rykersridgeblueberry

Summer Solstice Farms

Located in SE Indiana near Deputy, Indiana, Summer Solstice Farms raises dairy goats, chickens, Dexter cattle, and vegetables.

Products

Nigerian Dwarf Goats

Alpine Goats

Dexter Cattle

Free-Range Chicken Eggs (eating and hatching)

Summer Solstice Farms

(812) 873-8839

Land Line - no texts please

http://www.summersolsticefarms.weebly.com

summersolsticefarms@yahoo.com

Call or email to set visiting appointment

Jennings County

Clark's Berry Farm

The farm has been a family owned farm for over 100 years. Using integrated pest management, drip irrigation and cover crops, Clark's Berry Farm provides fresh picked fruit from June until August. Berries include strawberries, red and black raspberries, blueberries and blackberries. Customers can pick the berries themselves using Clark's containers, or purchase ready picked berries. Their berries have won top honors at the Indiana State Fair. Cash only.

Clark's Berry Farm

8905 W 350 S

North Vernon, IN 47265

(812) 344-5401

https://www.facebook.com/clarkberryfarm/

Collins Cove Greenhouse

Collins Cove Greenhouse is a locally owned greenhouse operation that offers a wide variety of plants, including vegetable plants, flowers, perennials and potted plants.

Collins Cove Greenhouse

5825 N In-3

North Vernon, Indiana 47265

Get Directions

North Vernon, IN

(812) 346-1973

https://www.facebook.com/Collins-Cove-Greenhouse-103398906364853/?rf=1608792339408897

Marion's Greenhouse

We have owned the greenhouse since 2004; it was in operation for 15 years prior as well. We also have a full retail gift shop, including garden decor and garden pharmaceuticals, etc. pots, planters, concrete statuary, along with soils, mulches, and fertilizers. We are well known for our unique planter combos, "Vintage Garden Designs", using old repurposed "junk" for garden planters and yard decor. Thank you for including us. Lorraine Henry

Marion's Greenhouse

4066 N State Road 3

Deputy, Indiana 47230

(812) 866-2856

https://www.facebook.com/Marionsgreenhouse/

New Creation Daylilies

New Creation Daylilies specializes in providing a wide selection of daylilies. The open dates vary per year, usually late June through early July. Call, email or check their Facebook page for current times and information.

New Creation Daylilies

Mark & Becky Eberts

1120 W State Hwy 250

Deputy, IN 47230

(in Old Paris)

812-592-3777

newcreationdaylilies@yahoo.com

www.newcreationdaylilies.com

https://www.facebook.com/New-Creation-Daylilies-329124916339/

North Vernon Farmers Market

Open April through October

7:30 a.m. to 1:00 p.m. Tuesday Thursday and Saturday

Located at the City Park in Shelter House #2

North Vernon Farmers Market

604 N State St

North Vernon, Indiana

(812) 346-9371

https://www.facebook.com/North-Vernon-Farmers-Market-1436311493354637/

Stream Cliff Herb Farm, Tea Room and Winery

Revolutionary War veteran James Harmon migrated into Jennings County, Indiana in 1821 to claim a land grant issued to pay the soldiers for their services during the war. Harmon, a bachelor, took up residence at first in a large hollow tree. He kept hogs in the base of the tree. The body heat generated by the hogs kept his abode warm. He constructed a barn and a home from bricks he baked himself during the 1820's and 1830's. General John Hunt Morgan's troops passed through the farm during their famous raid through southern Indiana in July, 1863. Mr. Harmon passed away a few month's later, in October. Harmon had never married and willed the farm to Asbury College, which established the Harmon Chair for Professorship of Biblical Literacy in his honor. Mr. Harmon is interred in a nearby cemetery.

Current Owners

The current owners, Gerald and Betty Manning, established the business over 40 years ago. Mrs. Mannings great grandfather purchased the farm from the Methodist Church, thus the farm has been in the family for five generations. The Mannings began by selling crafts, handmade blacksmith items, cornhusks dolls, dried florals and hand-carved Santa Clause figures. The business has thrived and currently offers wine made on the farm, a greenhouse/nursery, herbs, and teas. The family also operates the Twigs & Sprigs Restaurant and a gift shop.

Stream Cliff Herb Farm

8225 CR 90 W

Commiskey, IN 47227

http://www.streamclifffarm.com

https://www.facebook.com/Stream-Cliff-Farm-Restaurant-Winery-134812993240947/

Jennings County Visitors & Recreation Commission

Box 215

Vernon IN 47282

http://www.jenningsco.org

Ohio County

Rising Sun Farmers' Market

Rising Sun Farmers' Market

Historic Main Street

The public is invited to downtown Rising Sun, Ind. for the annual Farmer's Market each Saturday morning beginning at 9:00 a.m. mid-June throughout the growing season.

Held on Historic Main Street, products will include fresh local fruits and vegetables, honey, craft items, wood carvings, handmade jewelry and more!

The market is located on 211 Main Street in Rising Sun in front of Smoke on the Water Tobacco and Café/Roger That Cell Phone and Tablet Repair

103 S. Walnut St.

Rising Sun, IN 47040

Late April-October

Saturdays: 8:30 a.m.-Noon

https://www.facebook.com/events/1413149918702569/

Ohio County/Rising Sun Tourism

100 S. Walnut St.

Rising Sun, IN 47040

http://enjoyrisingsun.com/

812-438-4933

Ripley County

Batesville Farmers Market

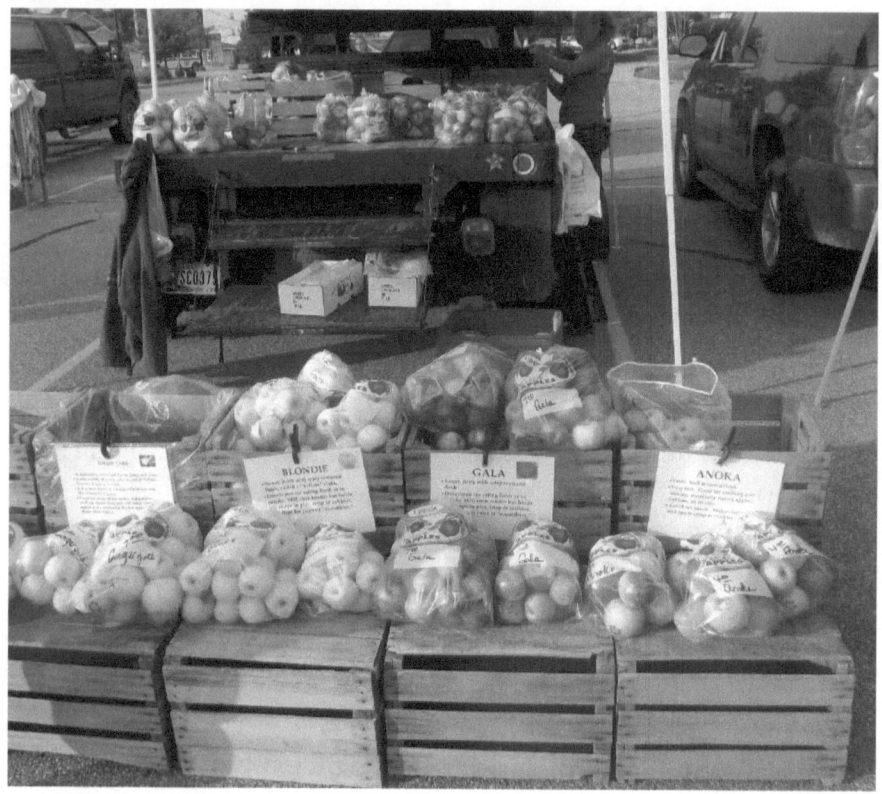

Established in 2002, the Batesville Farmers Market strives to provide locally grown food by local farmers in the freshest form possible. The market opens in May and remains open on Saturdays from 8:00 - 11:00 AM every Saturday.

Batesville Farmers Market

George Street

Batesville, IN 47006

https://www.facebook.com/BatesvilleFarmersMarket/

batesvillefarmersmarket@hotmail.com

Beaver Creek Nursery

Founded in 1999, Beaver Creek Nursery offers a wide variety of plants and services. The largest retail nursery in Indiana the product line includes over 400 varieties of trees, shrubs, ornamentals, perennials, topiaries and miniatures. Beaver Creek grows many of their trees, shrubs and perennials in containers, which allows customers the convenience of taking them home to plant. Gardeners may plant container grown stock at any time of year. Beaver Creek operates a "test plot," where they test new varieties to check their hardiness in this area.

Fountains and Ponds

Beaver Creek also stocks pond and waterfall construction supplies. They can build your fountain, pond or waterfall or teach you how to do it yourself.

Landscaping and Hard Scape

Beaver Creek also provides a full range of landscaping design and installation services. They also stock patio and retaining wall blocks as well as stone, gravel and mulches. They also provide wholesale pricing for businesses.

Beaver Creek Nursery

5530 West County Rd - 900 South

Madison, IN 47250

812-689-5595

http://beavercreeknurseryin.com

Dots Bulk Foods

Founded by Aaron and Kate Nobbe in 2007, Dot's Bulk Foods offers a wide variety of specialty and bulk food products.

Their extensive product line includes:

Homemade fudge made fresh in house with real butter

Old fashioned candies

Snacks

Nuts

Dried fruits

Pasta

Jams & jellies

Soups

Baking mixes

Flavorings & oils

Organic & dietary foods

Peanut & almond butters with no oils or additives

Frozen fruits

Organic, grass-fed buffalo & beef

Baking supplies – cookie cutters, cake boxes, etc.

Gifts

Dots Bulk Foods

394 Northside Dr.

Batesville, IN 47006

dottysbulkfoodbasket@gmail.com

http://www.dottysbulkfood.com

https://www.facebook.com/dottysbulkfoods

Five Oaks Garden Center

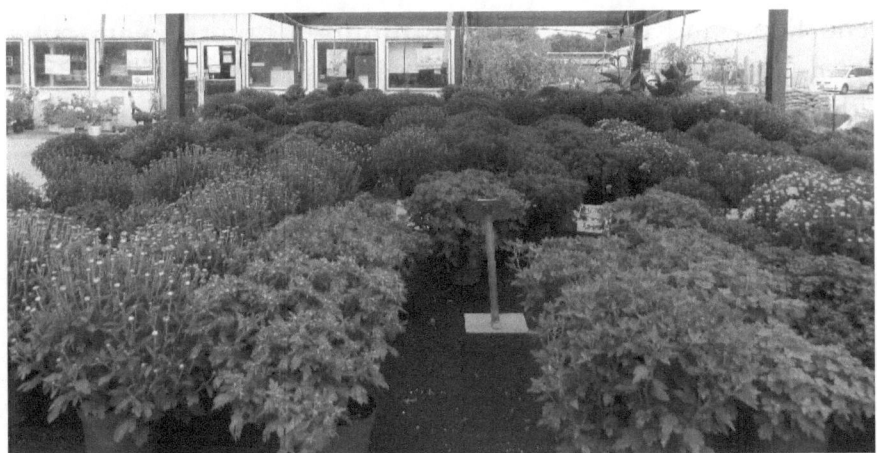

Matt and Marla Nobbe established Five Oaks Garden Center in 1989 with one greenhouse. Over the years the operation has grown to eight greenhouses and two acres of nursery stock. Five Oaks produces their own plants, their selection including many varieties of vegetables, annual, perennial and herb plants. In the garden center they stock a full selection of garden supplies like fertilizers, pesticides, tools and other gardening necessities. The store also offers a nice line of gardening oriented gift items. Gardeners will also find a great selection of fall mums, pansies and ornamental cabbages during the early autumn months. They also sell pumpkins, gourds and scarecrows in their garden center.

Five Oaks Garden Center

279 State Road 129 South

Batesville, IN 47006

http://www.fiveoaksgarden.com/

https://www.facebook.com/5OaksGardenCenter/

(812) 934-3625

5oaks@etczone.com

Food and Growers Association

The Food and Growers Association endeavors to promote local food production in the Laughery Valley area via education and networking. The Association sponsors an annual conference for growers and consumers.

A Short History of the Food and Growers Association by the Author

Summarized by Information Provided by Deanna Hookway

The vision to create a locally produced food system for consumers by founders Geralyn Litzinger, dietitians Kathy Cooley and Kyle Thompson with Sister Claire Whalen began in 2004. A meeting by the group in November 2004 produced a plan to utilize two existing programs, the Share the Bounty Program and the Batesville Farmers' Market to form the nucleus of a new organization that would:

Advance the health in our community through healthy-eating opportunities

Offer an economic stimulus for family farmers by creating a safe and secure local food source

Promote agri-tourism in the geographic region that included Batesville/Oldenburg and the Laughery Valley region's farms and towns

Share the Bounty Program

The Share the Bounty Program is a program operated by Micala Farm in Oldenburg that distributes fresh, locally grown food to low income people in Batesville and the Oldenburg area. The Program offers a twice weekly nutritional program that recipients must take to remain eligible for the program. Formed in 2002, the Share the Bounty Program has operated annually since its founding.

Vision to Reality

The founders of the Food and Growers Association of Laughery Valley and its Environs began the work of organizing the organization's network at a meeting in November 2005. Others in the area interested in the new organization met in November to draft a mission statement, established goals and wrote the organization's bylaws and articles of incorporation. Members of the group suggested a name change to the Food and Growers Association. They developed a web site, launched in July 2006 and had the Batesville Farmers Market established as a regular weekly event. The same year the FGA established its Community Supported Agriculture (CSA) project, with the goal of providing a market for area growers. The group began sponsoring an educational seminar in February 2007, an event which has become an annual event.

Community Supported Agriculture

Consumers interested in buying locally produced foods may purchase shares from a local CSA the CSA then provides the customer with a "box" of fresh vegetables and/or other locally produced agricultural products. This food is distributed throughout the growing season.

For more information, contact:

Food and Growers Association

c/o Deanna Hookway

1032 3 Mile Rd

Batesville, IN 47006

http://www.foodandgrowers.org

http://www.facebook.com/pages/Food-and-Growers-Association-of-Laughery-Valley/173766386057890

Garden Shack

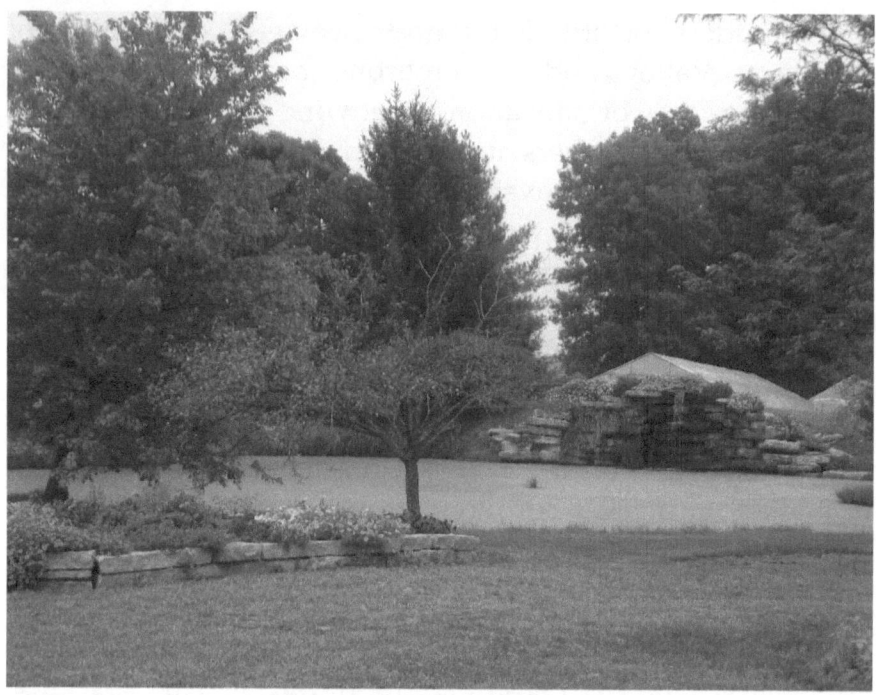

The garden shack has grown from its beginning in 1974 as a farm raising cows, pigs and corn. In 1980 the family added vegetables, fruits and melons they grew on their farm. The family sold its produce in Cincinnati. They used damaged crops to feed their animals and used the fertilizer the animals produced to fertilize the fields. By 1895 they began growing flowers in 1905 and opened their Batesville location in 1989. They opened a new location in 2006 in Milford, fifteen minutes from downtown Cincinnati. The Garden Shack sells vegetable transplants, bedding plants, perennial flowers, vegetables, pumpkins and fall mums at their retail stores and at various farmers markets around the area.

Garden Shack

5757 Hwy 46

Batesville, Indiana 47006

812-933-1155

Garden Shack

222 Wooster Pike

Milford, Ohio 45150

513-831-0517

https://oldegardenshack.com/

https://www.facebook.com/thegardenandbeachshack/

Greene Pastures

Greene Pastures sells goat milk, soaps, and Lotions

Greene Pastures

8536 W US Highway 50

Holton IN, 47023

765-546-8919

cagreenpastures@gmail.com

Kestler Farms

Kestler Farms raises Angus cattle using no antibiotics or hormones. They utilize a six month feeding program culminating with a final grain feeding period. After slaughtering Kestler Farms dry ages the meat, which produces a tender, juicy, flavorful beef. Customers may purchase individual cuts like roasts and steaks, or in bulk by purchasing by the quarter, half or whole.

Kestler Farms

1-812-934-4835

info@kestlerfarms.com

http://www.kestlerfarms.com/

https://www.facebook.com/bestbeefchoice/

Meyer's Produce

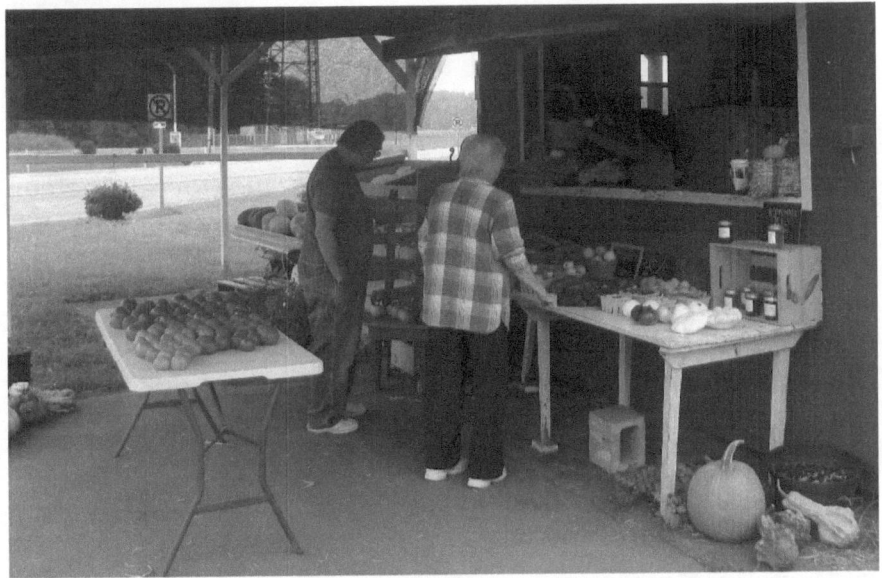

Meyer's Produce sells fresh vegetables from a roadside stand at the corner of Indiana State Roads 101 and 46.

Their fresh local produce includes watermelon, cantaloupe, tomatoes, cucumbers, sweet corn, pumpkins, gourds, and many other vegetables.

Meyer's Produce sets up at Batesville, Greensburg, and Brookville farmers markets every week. Just look for the big red truck!

Penntown, Indiana 47041

(812) 209-9217

https://www.facebook.com/meyersproducefarm/

Pat's Bulk Foods

Established in 1990 as an Amish style bulk food store, Pat's Bulk Foods has established a customer base that includes visitors from Indiana, Ohio and Kentucky. The store began as Welch's Grocery in the 1920's. The store offers an extensive line of baking goods that includes nineteen different kinds of flour, spices, nuts, grains, pastas, homemade nut butters, raw local honey, Amish jams and jellies, meat cures & seasonings, Bragg's vinegars, and frozen food items. They have Indiana grown beef, pork and chickens as well as many other food items produced in the state.

Pat's Bulk Foods

4492 US-421

Versailles, IN 47042

https://patsbulkfoods.com

https://www.facebook.com/PatsBulkFood/

Patterson Nursery

Customers will have an almost botanical garden experience when they visit Patterson Nursery, located on Michigan Road south of Holton Indiana. The nursery offers an ample choice of perennials, trees, shrubs and mulches. Patterson's also sells vegetable transplants, balled and burlapped nursery stock and herbs in their greenhouses.

Over 40 years of Horticulture experience.

Degreed and Certified Horticulturist

Award winning landscape installation

Pesticide licensed

Turf application licensed

We create outdoor living spaces

Landscape design and Installation

Commercial , Residential & Municipal

Complete Grounds Maintenance.

Sod Installation

Paver Walkways

Landscape Design / Build

Tree and Shrub Installation

Hardscape Walkways.

Paver Patios

Landscape Lighting

Natural Stone Walls

Flagstone Patios

Aquascape Installation

Retaining Wall Installation

Floral Design

Turf Fertilization / Weed Control

Lawn Renovation / Seed / Sod.

Patterson Nursery

2940 S. Old Michigan Road

Holton, Indiana 47023

812-689-0102

http://www.pattersonsnursery.com

Ripley County Farmers Market

305 Buckeye St.

Osgood, IN 47034

(812) 689-4718

305 Buckeye St., Osgood, IN 47037

https://ripleycountytourism.com/business-directory/701/ripley-county-farmers-market/

Sheets Tree Farm

A family farm owned by the same family since 1854, the farm originally comprised 40 acres. The farm has since expanded to 140, 35 of which are planted in Christmas Trees. Gayle and Lenna Sheets first planted the trees in the 1950's and opened the Choose & Cut Christmas Tree Farm about ten years later. In 1968 the farm supplied the White House with the Christmas Tree. For information about the farm's seasonal hours, check the website.

Types of Trees

Canaan Fir

Colorado Spruce

Norway Spruce

Scotch Pine

White Pine

Sheets Tree Farm

5679 N Co Rd 200 E

 Osgood, IN 47037

https://sheetstreefarm.com

Versailles Market on the Square Farmers Market

Sponsored by Main Street Versailles the Market opens in late May to early June and remains open until late September from 9:00 AM to 1:00 PM. Main Street Versailles formed on January 1, 2015 to create events and a positive interest to downtown Versailles.

Located on the Ripley County Courthouse Square

Saturdays 9am-1pm

May 28th-Sep 17

Versailles Market on the Square Farmers Market

101 E 1st North St

Courthouse Square

Versailles, IN 47042

Website: Market on the Square

(512) 937-4228

We accept SNAP, FMNP, debit/credit card

https://www.facebook.com/mainstreetversailles/

mainstreetversailles@gmail.com

Vogt's Farm

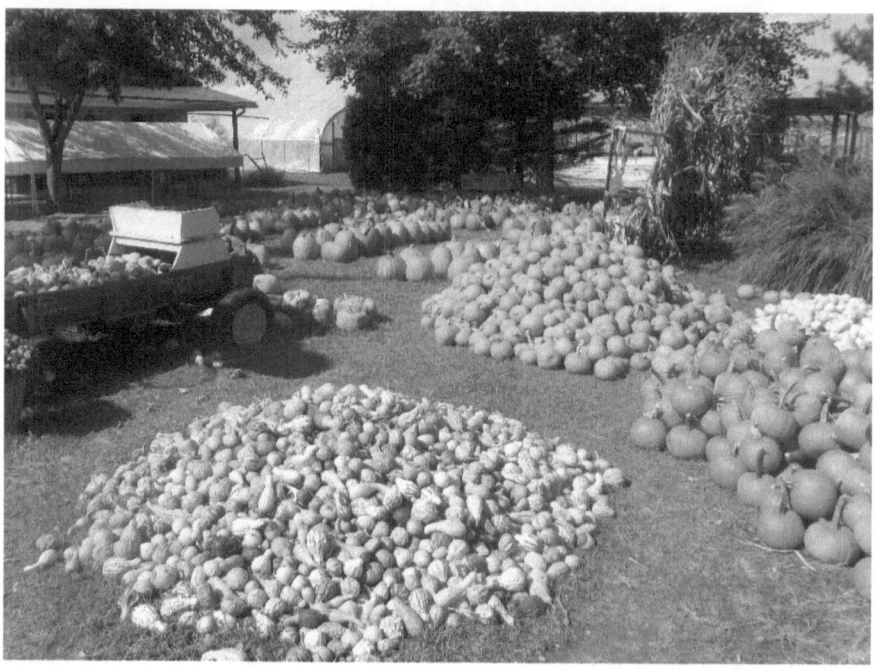

Visitors to Vogt's Farm will find a small, family farm that offers vegetable and flower transplants for sale in the spring, bluberries in June and the Pumpkin Festival in the fall. Customers may ride a horse drawn trolley to the pumpkin patch and pick a pumpkin from the field. They can also enjoy homemade pumpkin pie, pumpkin bread and pumpkin rolls and participate in many fun family oriented activities.

Vogt's Farm

12115 N State Road 129

Batesville, IN 47006

(812) 934-4627

https://www.facebook.com/pg/vogtfarmbatesville

Weber Greenhouses

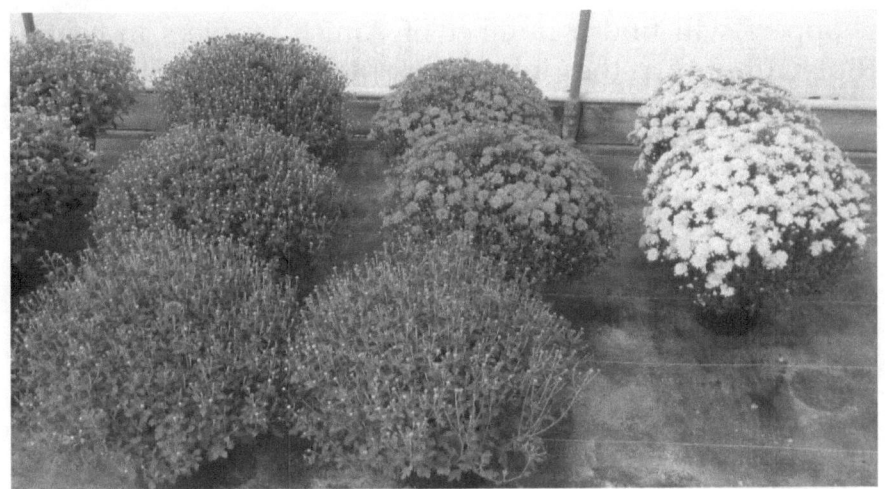

Weber Greenhouses offers wholesale and retail bedding plants, vegetable transplants, chrysanthemums and more.

Weber Greenhouses

701 N. Meridian Street

Sunman IN, 47041

812-623-3216

webersgreenhouse@etczone.com

Ripley County Tourism Bureau

PO Box 21   220 East US 50

Versailles, IN 47042

http://www.ripleycountytourism.com/

812-689-7431

Amish Growers

Shoppers will find a number of Amish growers in central Ripley County in the Holton area. Most of these growers are open to the public and many sell their products at local farmer's Markets.

Levi Beiler Jr.

4991 West County Road 550 S

Holton, Indiana 47023

812-689-6891

Mums

Produce

Rose Plants - Potted

Sadie Bieleer

4909 W. County Road 550 S

Holton, IN 47023

812-689-6598

Vegetable Plants

Greenhouse

Flowers

Benjamin Smoker

8499 South Old Michigan Road

Madison, Indiana

812-621-4094

Perennials

Produce

Jesse Stoltzfus

812-689-6834

Bulk Food Store

Produce

Mums

Strawberries

Greenhouse

Samuel Stolzfus

812-756-3077

Produce

Greenhouse

Country Creations

6851 S. US 421

Versaille, IN

812-689-4243

Baked Shop

Deli

Produce

David Stoltzfus

S-Curve Greenhouse

4312 West County Road 450 South

Holton, IN 47023

812-689-6013

Mums

Pumpkins

Strawberries

Rolling Acres Greenhouse

Joel and Malinda Stoltzfus

4634 W County Road 600S

Holton, IN 47023

812-621-8953

Vegetables

Flowers

Produce

Pumpkin

Yellow Winter Squash

Samuel Stoltzfus

4925 W County Road 550 S

Holton, IN 47023

812-756-4131

Strawberries

Blackberries

Raspberries

Scott County

Arbuckle Greenhouses

Established in 1995, Arbuckle Greenhouses produces an extensive line of annual flowers, vegetables and many other flowering plant products at their family owned greenhouse in Scottsburg. They are also a wholesale grower of growing plugs and liners for area greenhouses.

Arbuckle Greenhouses

1292 W Leota Rd

Scottsburg, IN 47170

http://arbucklegreenhouses.com/index.html

https://www.facebook.com/Arbuckles-Greenhouse-415373535480747/?rf=110403032357878

Robbins Farm and Nursery

Robbins Farm and Nursery produces a large selection of Christmas trees available during the Christmas holiday season as well as nursery stock available year round.

Shrubs include:

Boxwood

Arborvitae

Japanese Maple

Crabapples

Bradford Pears

Japanese Yews

Christmas Products include:

Christmas Wreaths

Frasier Fir

White Pine

Various Spruce Species

Scotch Pine

All Christmas trees also available as balled and burlapped nursery stock, ready for planting.

Robbins Farm and Nursery

3278 West Lake Road

Scottsburg, Indiana 47170

(812) 820-1146

https://robbins.farm/

robbinsfarmnursery@gmail.com

https://www.facebook.com/RobbinsNurseryFarm/

Scott County Farmers' Market

Location:

Scottsburg Heritage Station Train Depot parking lot in Scottsburg, Indiana

Saturdays, 8 AM - noon

Thursdays, noon – 5PM

May - October

Contact:

Scott County Farmers' Market

90 North Main Street

Scottsburg, Indiana

812-701-6460

https://www.facebook.com/scottcountyfarmersmarket/

Switzerland County

Center Square Discount

Amish owned & operated. Groceries, bulk foods, Amish crafts, & fresh produce. Center Square Discount offers a large selection of cheeses, dairy products and seasonal fruit. The market is located on State Road 56 in Vevay's Center Square.

8 AM – 6 PM Monday-Friday, Saturday, 8 AM – 3 PM

Center Square Discount

1722 Hwy 56 (Center Square),

Vevay, IN 47043

Telephone:

812-427-2594

https://switzcotourism.com/item/center-square-discount/

Switzerland County Farmers and Artisans Marketplace

Downtown, Vevay, IN, 47043

On the corner of Main Cross Street and Main Street, farmers and artisans are encouraged to sell their produce, livestock, artistic items, and more. Every Saturday morning May through November.

Switzerland County Farmers and Artisans Marketplace

https://www.facebook.com/Switzerland-County-Farmers-and-Artisans-Marketplace-649252595102544/

Switzerland County Tourism
128 W Main Street
Vevay IN 47043
http://www.switzcotourism.com/
800-435-5688

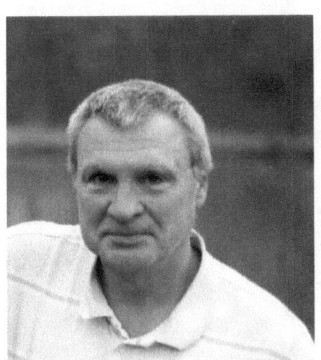

About the Author

Paul considers himself a bit of an Indiana hound, in that he likes to sniff out the interesting places and history of Indiana and use his books to tell people about them.

Join Paul on Facebook
https://www.facebook.com/Mossy-Feet-Books-474924602565571/
Twitter
https://twitter.com/MossyFeetBooks
mossyfeetbooks@gmail.com

Mossy Feet Books Catalog

To Get Your Free Copy of the Mossy Feet Books Catalogue, Click This Link.

http://mossyfeetbooks.blogspot.com/

Gardening Books

Fantasy Books

Humor

Science Fiction

Semi – Autobiographical Books

Travel Books

Sample Chapter

The Agricultural and 4-H Fair - Southeast Edition

Dearborn County Fair

The Dearborn County Agricultural Society formed on April 10, 1852 with Seth Platt as president. The association held the first Dearborn County Fair in Manchester on October 27, 28, 29, 1852. . The expenses for the fair totaled $113.00 and gate the fair's gate receipts were $261.75. This fair was successful, and encouraged the sponsors to raise ticket prices. The fair remained in Manchester until 1856 when the Society leased nine acres of land shaded by a grove of sugar maple trees in Aurora. This property is now the Aurora City Park. The circular drive was originally a race track.

Rivalry Ensues

Two years later a rivalry between Aurora and Lawrenceburg arose over which should host the county fair. The first classes began and included sheep, cattle, hogs, and poultry. The home Economics portion included instructions on jelly making, fruit butters, pickles, baking, and needlework. Both cities held fairs in 1858, a situation that would continue until 1869, when the Lawrenceburg Agriculture Association formed and the fair moved to Lawrenceburg.

Lawrenceburg Agricultural Association

Lawrenceburg Agricultural Association formed in 1879 and held their first fair on the old fairgrounds in 1880 at the end of Center Street. They later purchased 8 across which allowed them to construct a 1/2 mile race track, which gained the reputation as the finest in the country. The grandstand held 2500 people it rained every day during this fair, however attendance was still good

Fire and Flood

In 1881 and again in 1882 fire destroyed the fairground and building.

The board rebuilt the fairground, which a flood promptly destroyed in 1883

The board rebuilt 48 stalls, the barn and fine art hall in time for the fair

Events and Programs

An example of some of the programs from the 1883 Dearborn County Fair Program:

Gus Sun Rodeo

Tumbling Arabs

The Singing Cowboys

Goat Races

Doll Baby Parade

Baby Show

Lamy's Height Casting Act

Rio Grande Rangers

Ramond's Contortion Act

Rajah Troupe

The admission was 25 cents.

Visitors could also inspect a Case farm tractor exhibit. A company representative was in attendance to conduct demonstrations and answer questions. Equipment included tractors, cultivators, hay loaders and manure spreaders.

Goats and Roosters

During the goat race, the goats were hitched to carts driven by young boys. The fairground was near the Ohio River.

Another popular event was a Rooster Corn Eating Contest. The rooster that consumed the most corn during the contest won a prize for its boy or girl owner.

Victor Oberting sponsored parades with goats, horses, dogs and entertainers.

A nurse was in attendance at the rest rooms

Visitors got their drinking water from the town pump, used a tin cup.

Lawrenceburg Fair Association

In 1890 the Lawrenceburg Agricultural Society transferred ownership to the Lawrenceburg Fair Association. The Association took a ten year lease on the fairgrounds.

Fairs Discontinued

Lawrenceburg had no fair for eight years - 1882 - 1890

The Lawrenceburg Fair Association formed in 1890 and ran fairs for eighteen years

1894 Lawrenceburg Fair

August 22 - 25

Dearborn County had constructed a horse racing track that led the Chicago Times to announce, "Racing by fast steppers on the finest half mile track in the state." The Times stated that they would announce the fair activities at a later date. During this era railroads and river boats offered special excursion rates out to the county fairs in rural communities.

Fair activates included:

Balloon Races

Bicycle Races

Horse racing, including trotting and running

In addition there were fruit, vegetable and flower displays from local farmers.

1897 Fair

From a Fair Program for the August 26 1897 Fair

Cooks Mammoth Hippodrome

Riderless Horse Race

Steeple Chase Race

Standing Jockey Race

Bucking Horses

Chariot Races

Hurdle Races

Hound VS Horse Race

Running Team Race

Roman Standing Race

Harrison Fair

In 1897 Harrison organized its own fair, which they held in West Harrison for three years. A flood of the Whitewater River damaged the fairgrounds and the fair abandoned.

Cleaning up the Fair

Indianapolis News reported on October 25, 1898:

The Lawrenceburg Fair Board sold the fairgrounds to Victor Oberting, owner of the Garnier Oberting Brewing Company. The fair had been profitable when "hoochie coochie shows ran during the fair on the fairgrounds. An attempt by Oberting to clean up the fair resulted in a financial loss, leading Oberting to sell his shares, after which the fair would resume its previous programs.

Reported by theAngola Herald August 27, 1902, page 13:

The Lawrenceburg Fair Association formed in 1890 with William H. O'Brien as president, Victor Oberting as vice president.

Fair attendance averaged 12,000 - 15,000 and took in between $2000 - $2400 in ticket sales. The city owned the fairgrounds, which found use as a park during the time the fair was not in session.

The 1902 Dearborn County Fair Program included

Dearborn County Rough Riders Parade with 10 companies of Rough Riders

The 2000 troops would reenact the Battle of San Juan Hill

A military band also performed

Annie Oakley

Buckskin Ben

Note - the Rough Riders organized in Boon County, Kentucky and Dearborn County with Jacob Spanagel Barret commander

1903 Fair

The featured product at this fair was an interchangeable buggy and road wagons.

1908 Fair

1908 fair attendance was 15,000 people. Street cars bound from Harrison and Aurora were so full that men hung from the cow catchers on the front and rear of the cars.

There were no fairs during 1918, 1919, and 1920 due to World War I and the flu epidemic that followed.

1922 – Fair Resumes - August 23 - 26

1922 fair admission 50 cents

American Legion members free

1/2 mile mule race

County Road Race

Baby show

Horse races - most purses $200

Prizes awarded for the best

Vegetables,

Horse

Beef

Hog

Reported in the July 28, 1934 Dearborn County Register:

Congress of Daredevils

Famous Actress Crashes through wall

Feature of Thrill Day

Stock car driven 40 MPH into a wall

Mary Wiggins actress to participate in the crash

40,000 expected attendance

Ash Can Derby

Car Jump with Motorcycles

Rain Insurance Policy Expired July 28, 1934

Insurance Company of North America

The company insured gate receipts loss from 1/10 inch of rain or more also against sleet, hail and snow. The premium cost $63.60.

Reported in the July 19, 1937 Dearborn County Register

The newspaper reported extensive flood damage from the Ohio River flood that year. The Secretary Building was gone, the Auto Shed had collapsed, the art building twisted and wrecked, the horse tables damaged.

Forced Relocation

Levee construction in 1941 took most of the fairground, forcing its relocation to its current location. Governor Shricker attended the dedication ceremony and gave an address. Thunderstorms cut the crowd size down.

1952 Billboard Magazine

In 1952 Billboard Magazine selected the Dearborn County Fair as a typical county fair, Mrs. America visited the fair.

Activities during this period included:

Skating Smith - act included skating through a fifteen inch tunnel

Pat and Will Levold Equilibrists

Americas Greatest Slack Wire

Daily Aeroplane rides

Amusement Rides

Moral and Refined Entertainment

Fireworks - different show every night

Famous Savilla Trio

Acrobats

Comedians

Cotton Picking Trio

Dearborn County Band

5 horse races daily

1971 Amos Oberting organizes the Dog Show

1994 Abner Hall constructed

On June 24, 2002, the Lawrenceburg Journal Press reported:

A 2 million dollar renovation project included a speedway, grandstand and concession stand along with some other renovations

The Modern Fair

The modern Dearborn County Fair has evolved into a fair that highlights the many talents of young 4-H students. The fair also features a number of traditional events that include tractor pulls, a queen contest, fashion review and other fun activities. The event list currently includes:

4-H Poultry Show

4-H Dog Show

Youth Livestock Judging Contest

Opening Ceremony

Frog Jump Contest

Poultry Cooking Demo

4-H Royalty Crowning

Blue Grass Tractor Show

4-H Rabbit Show

Demonstration and Public Speaking

Contest Read Creative Writing

]4-H Fashion Review

Robotics and 3D Printing Demo

Flower Show

1-2-3-4 Kids Cook

Pedal Tractor Pull

4-H Swine Show

Lawn Mower Race and Back Seat Driver Race

Pygmy Fiber Class and Dairy Goat Show

Pike Bake Off

Baby Contest

Peach Baking Contest

Lamb Cooking Demo

Fun Horse Show

4-H Sheep Show

4-H Horse and Pony Show

Small Animal Supreme Showmanship Contest

4-H Pocket Pet Show

Cat Show

Lawn and Garden Contest

Alpaca and Llama Show

Dairy Show

4-H Beef Heifer Show

4-H Market Beef Show

Steam Powered Recycling

Muddy Madness - Kids games in the mud

Beef Cooking Demo - Marcia Parcell

Pig in the Pen

4-H Pork Chop Dinner

4-H Livestock Sale

Rodeo

The 4-H Program list for Dearborn County includes the following topics:

Beef

Cats

Dairy

Dog

Goats

Horse & Pony

Llama/Alpaca

Pocket Pets

Poultry

Game Bird Division

Duck Division

Turkey Division

Poultry Illustrated

Talk

Rabbit

Sheep

Swine

Aerospace

Alfalfa

Aquatic Science

Arts

& Crafts, Model Building and Wearable Arts

Beekeeping

Bicycle

Cake Decorating

Cat Poster

Child Development

Collections

Computers

Consumer Clothing

Consumer Dairy

Consumer Meats (Pork, Beef, & Lamb)

Corn

Creative Writing

Dog Poster

Electric

Entomology

Fashion Revue

Floriculture

-Flowers

Foods

Forestry

Frugal Fashion

Garden

Genealogy

Geology

Gift Wrapping

Hay

Health

Home Environment

Horse Science

Junior Leaders

Lawn & Garden Tractor

Llama/Alpaca Poster/Craft

People In My World

Photography

Potato

Poultry Display Boards/Science Display

Rabbit Poster

Radio

Recycling - Repurposing Project

Recycling Science Fair Project

Robotics

Scrapbook

Sewing

Sewing For Fun and Others

Shooting Sports

Small Grains (Barley, Oats, Rye, Triticale, Wheat)

Small Engines

Soil & Water Conservation

Soybeans

Sport fishing

Sports

Strawberry

Tobacco

Tractor

Veterinary Science

Weather

Weeds

Welding-Electric Arc

Wildlife

Woodworking

Dearborn County Fairground

351 E Eads Pkwy

Lawrenceburg, IN 47025

812-926-1189

https://www.dearborncounty4h.com/

https://www.facebook.com/DearbornCounty4HandCommunityFair/

Extension Office

812-926-1189

dearborncountyfair@yahoo.com

http://www.dearborncountyfair.com

https://extension.purdue.edu/Dearborn/pages/default.aspx

Mossy Feet Books
www.mossyfeetbooks.com

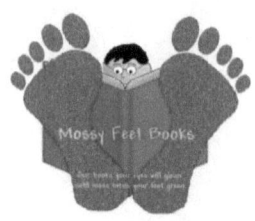